VAGINA CANCER

PREVENTIVE TECHNIQUES FOR VAGINA CANCER

DR. KATE .P

Contents

CHAPTER ONE

INTRODUCTION

Vaginal cancer is an uncommon type of cancer that develops in the muscular tube that joins your uterus to your external genitalia. The cells lining your vagina, also known as the birth canal, are most frequently the site of vaginal cancer.

Primary vaginal cancer is an uncommon kind of cancer that starts in your vagina, while many cancers can migrate from other parts of your body to your vagina.

The best chance of recovery is for women who have vaginal cancer in its early stages. Treatment for vaginal cancer that has spread outside the vagina is far more challenging.

Symptoms

It's possible that early vaginal cancer doesn't show any symptoms. Vaginal cancer may exhibit the following signs and symptoms as it advances:

unusual vaginal bleeding, such as that which occurs after menopause or after sexual activity

vaginal discharge that is wet

a growth or bump inside your vagina

painful urination

Constipation

Pelvic discomfort

When to visit a physician

If you experience any abnormal vaginal bleeding or other signs and symptoms associated with vaginal cancer, consult your physician. As symptoms and indicators of vaginal cancer are not always present, it is important to follow your doctor's advice regarding when to schedule routine pelvic checks.

Reasons

The cause of vaginal cancer is unknown. Generally speaking, cancer starts when normal cells become aberrant due to a genetic mutation that occurs in healthy cells.

Healthy cells divide and expand at a predetermined rate, dying at a predetermined age. Cancer cells don't die; instead, they proliferate and expand out of control. The aberrant cells build up to form a mass known as a tumor.

Cancer cells can split off from an original tumor and infiltrate neighboring tissues, dispersing throughout the body (metastasis).

Vaginal cancer types

Several forms of vaginal cancer can be distinguished according to the type of cell in which the disease first appeared. Types of vaginal cancer include:

The most prevalent kind of vaginal squamous cell carcinoma starts in the thin, flat cells (squamous cells) that line the surface of the vagina.

Vaginal adenocarcinoma is a cancer that starts in the glandular cells that line your vagina.

The pigment-producing cells (melanocytes) in your vagina produce vaginal melanoma.

Vaginal sarcoma is a cancer that arises in the muscles or connective tissue cells that line your vagina.

RISK ELEMENTS

The following are some factors that could raise your risk of vaginal cancer:

growing older. As you become older, your chance of vaginal cancer rises. The majority of women diagnosed with vaginal cancer are over 60 years old.

Vaginal intraepithelial neoplasia is the term for abnormal cells seen in the vagina. The risk of vaginal cancer is higher in women who have vaginal intraepithelial neoplasia (VAIN).

Vaginal cells in women with VAIN appear different from normal cells, but not enough different to be classified as cancerous. Though doctors are unsure of what causes some cases to evolve into cancer and others to remain benign, a small percentage of women with VAIN will eventually acquire vaginal cancer.

The sexually transmitted human papillomavirus (HPV), which can also cause vulvar, cervical, and vaginal malignancies, is the source of VAIN. There are vaccines available that guard against some forms of HPV infection.

exposure to certain anti-miscarriage medications. Women who had moms who used diethylstilbestrol (DES) during pregnancy in the 1950s are more likely to develop clear cell adenocarcinoma, a specific kind of vaginal cancer.

Additional risk factors associated with an elevated risk of vaginal cancer include:

several partners for sex

Early years of first sexual encounters

Consuming tobacco

HIV infection

It is possible for vaginal cancer to metastasis, or spread, to other parts of your body such your liver, lungs, and bones.

Getting Ready for Your Consultation

If you see any symptoms or indicators that bother you, schedule a visit with a gynecologist or your family physician. In the event that vaginal cancer is diagnosed, you will probably be directed to a gynecologic oncologist, a medical professional who specializes in malignancies of the female reproductive system.

It's a good idea to be well prepared because appointments are often short and there's a lot of territory to cover. Here are some preparation tips for you and what to anticipate from your physician.

What you're capable of

Jot down any symptoms you're having, even if they don't seem to be connected to the reason you made the visit.

Important personal details, such as significant stressors or recent life transitions, should be included.

Enumerate every drug you take, including vitamins and supplements.

Invite a friend or member of your family to accompany you. It can occasionally be challenging to take in everything that is said during an appointment. It's possible that someone with you will recall something you overlooked or forgot.

Prepare a list of inquiries for your physician

Making the most of your time with your doctor can be achieved by organizing your questions in advance of your appointment. In the event that time runs out, prioritize your list of questions from most to least important. Some fundamental inquiries to make of your physician regarding vaginal cancer are:

Which of my symptoms is most likely to be the cause?

Are my symptoms coming from any other sources?

Which tests are necessary for me?

Which kinds of therapies are offered? Which side effects should I anticipate from each treatment? How will my sexuality be impacted by these treatments?

Which course of action do you believe is best for me?

What are the alternatives you propose to the main strategy?

These additional medical conditions affect me. How do I oversee them both the best I can?

Are there any rules that I have to abide by?

Has my cancer progressed? At what point in time is it?

Which way do I stand?

Must I consult a specialist? Will my insurance pay for that, and how much will it cost?

Can I bring brochures or any other printed materials with me? Which websites would you suggest?

During your consultation, feel free to ask questions as they come to mind in addition to the ones you have prepared in advance.

CHAPTER TWO

What to anticipate from your physician

You'll probably be asked a lot of questions by your doctor. It might help free up time for any other questions you might have if you're prepared to respond to them. Your physician might inquire:

When did you start feeling the effects?

Have you experienced constant symptoms or just sporadic ones?

What level of severity do you have?

What appears to alleviate your problems, if anything?

What seems to exacerbate your symptoms, if anything?

Are you aware if your mother used DES during her pregnancy?

Have you ever had cancer in your personal history?

Have you ever received a diagnosis of HPV?

Have you ever had a Pap test that was abnormal?

Exams and diagnosis

screening for vaginal cancer in healthy women

Sometimes vaginal cancer is discovered during a normal pelvic exam before symptoms show up.

A pelvic exam involves your doctor carefully examining your outer genitalia, feeling your uterus and ovaries with two fingers inserted into your vagina while pressing your belly with the other hand. Additionally, he or she places a speculum—a device—into your vagina. Your doctor can examine your vagina and cervix for anomalies when the speculum opens your vaginal canal.

Also, your doctor might perform a Pap test. Pap tests are typically used to check for cervical cancer, however they can also occasionally reveal the presence of vaginal cancer cells.

The frequency of these screenings is determined by your cancer risk factors and the existence of abnormal Pap tests in the past. Consult your physician about the recommended frequency of these exams.

Examinations to identify vaginal cancer

In order to look for anomalies that can point to vaginal cancer, your doctor might perform a Pap test and pelvic examination. In light of those results, your physician might carry out more tests to ascertain whether you have vaginal cancer, including:

examining the vagina under a magnifying glass. A colposcope, a specialized light-powered magnification tool, is used to examine your vagina during a colposcopy. During a colposcopy, your doctor can see any patches of abnormal cells on the surface of your vagina by magnifying it.

taking a sample of vaginal tissue so that it can be tested. A biopsy involves taking a sample of questionable tissue in order to look for cancerous cells. A biopsy of tissue may be taken by your doctor during a colposcopy examination. The tissue sample is sent by your doctor to a lab for analysis.

Setting Up

Following a vaginal cancer diagnosis, your doctor will stage the cancer to ascertain its exact location. Your doctor can determine the best course of therapy for you based on the stage of your cancer. Your doctor may use one of the following methods to assess the stage of your cancer:

imaging examinations. To find out if the cancer has spread, your doctor might prescribe imaging studies. MRIs, CT scans, positron emission tomography (PET), magnetic resonance imaging (MRI), and X-rays are examples of imaging examinations.

Your body can be seen through tiny cameras. Your doctor may be able to see if cancer has spread to specific places of your body with the use of procedures that utilize tiny cameras to see inside your body. During a cystoscopy or proctoscopy, cameras assist your doctor in viewing within your bladder and rectum.

Your cancer is given a stage after your doctor assesses its severity. Stages of cervical cancer include:

Stage I: Only the vaginal wall is affected by the cancer.

Stage II: The tissue adjacent to your vagina has been affected by cancer.

Stage III: The pelvis has been further penetrated by the cancer.

Stage IVA: The cancer has progressed to adjacent organs, like the rectum or bladder.

Stage IVB: The cancer has progressed to organs other than the vagina, like the liver.

The kind and stage of the vaginal cancer you have are among the many variables that affect your treatment options. Based on your treatment goals and the side effects you're ready to accept, you and your doctor collaborate to decide which treatments are ideal for you. Radiation and surgery are commonly used in the treatment of vaginal cancer.

Operation

Women with vaginal cancer may have any of the following surgical procedures:

Removal of tiny tumors or lesions. Cancer restricted to the surface of your vagina may be cut away, along with a small margin of surrounding healthy tissue to ensure that all of the cancer cells have been removed.

vaginal excision, or vaginectomy. It might be required to remove all of the cancer by either performing a radical vaginectomy or a partial vaginectomy, which involves removing portion of your vagina. Your surgeon may suggest a vaginectomy combined with a hysterectomy (removal of the uterus and ovaries) or a lymphadenectomy (removal of the adjacent lymph nodes) depending on the severity of your malignancy.

Pelvic exenteration is the removal of most of the pelvic organs. If your vaginal cancer has returned or if it has progressed throughout your pelvic region, then major surgery can be necessary. Many of the organs in your pelvic area, such as your bladder, ovaries, uterus, vagina, rectum, and the lower part of your colon, may be removed by the surgeon during pelvic exenteration. Your abdomen is made to have openings that let waste (colostomy) and urine (urostomy) leave your body and collect in ostomy bags.

Should your vagina be extracted entirely, you can decide to have a new vagina surgically created. To create a new vagina, surgeons may utilize flaps of muscle, fragments of skin, or portions of intestine from other parts of your body. You can engage in vaginal sex with a repaired vagina if you make certain modifications. But your own vagina isn't the same as a recreated one. For example, due to modifications in surrounding nerves, a reconstructed vagina lacks natural lubrication and produces a distinct sensation when touched.

Radiation treatment

High-powered energy beams, like X-rays, are used in radiation therapy to destroy cancer cells. There are two ways to administer radiation:

radiation from the outside. Depending on the severity of your cancer, external beam radiotherapy may target your pelvis alone or your entire abdomen. You lie on a table while a sizable radiation equipment moves around you to target the treatment area during external beam radiotherapy. Most vaginal cancer patients receive radiation therapy from an external beam.

radioactivity inside. Radioactive objects, such as seeds, wires, cylinders, or other materials, are inserted into your vagina or the surrounding tissue during internal radiation therapy, also known as brachytherapy. The devices might be taken out after a predetermined period of time. Internal radiation is the only treatment available to women with very early-stage vaginal cancer. After receiving external radiation, other women could get internal radiation.

Radiation therapy destroys rapidly proliferating cancer cells, but it can have unfavorable side effects by harming neighboring healthy cells.

Radiation side effects vary depending on the radiation's intensity and direction of impact.

Other choices

You could be offered additional therapies if radiation and surgery are unable to control your cancer, such as:

chemotherapy. Chemicals are used in chemotherapy to destroy cancer cells. The efficacy of chemotherapy in treating female vaginal cancer patients is unclear. Because of this, vaginal cancer is rarely treated with chemotherapy alone. Radiation therapy may be combined with chemotherapy to increase radiation's efficacy.

CHAPTER THREE

clinical examinations. Clinical trials are studies done to evaluate novel therapeutic approaches. A cure is not guaranteed, but participating in a clinical study allows you to try the newest advancements in treatment. To learn more about your possibilities, talk with your doctor about the clinical trials that are now accepting participants.

WAY OF LIFE AND DOMESTIC MEDICINE

It is impossible to completely avoid vaginal cancer. Nonetheless, you could lower your risk if you:

Get Pap testing and pelvic checks on a regular basis. Regular pelvic exams and Pap testing can help to increase the likelihood that vaginal cancer is detected early. Early detection increases the likelihood of vaginal cancer recovery. Talk to your doctor about the best time to start these tests and how frequently to do them.

Consult your physician about the HPV vaccination. Getting vaccinated against HPV can lower your risk of developing vaginal cancer and other malignancies linked to HPV. Find out from your doctor if getting the HPV vaccine is right for you.

Avoid smoking. Give up smoking if you do. Don't start if you don't smoke. Vaginal cancer is more likely to occur in smokers.

Adapting and providing assistance

Every woman with cancer responds differently to her diagnosis. To process your emotions, you might wish to spend time with friends and family or request some alone time. Your diagnosis may have left you feeling disoriented and insecure about who you are. To aid in your coping, attempt:

Have adequate knowledge about your cancer to decide how best to be treated. Make a list of the inquiries you want to make when you see your doctor next. Invite a family member or friend to accompany you to appointments so they may take notes. Find out more information sources from your medical team. When it comes time to choose your course of therapy, you could feel better at ease if you have greater knowledge regarding your illness.

Continue to be intimate with your spouse. Treatments for vaginal cancer may have side effects that make it harder for you and your partner to have intimate sexual relations. Try to come up with new strategies for preserving intimacy if your treatment makes having sex uncomfortable or impractical. Having deep conversations and spending quality time together are two strategies to increase your emotional connectedness. Take your time getting intimate when you're ready. Speak with your doctor if the sexual side effects of your cancer therapy are causing problems in your relationship with your spouse. In addition to referring you to a professional, he or she might advise coping mechanisms for sexual adverse effects.

Establish a network of support. Support from friends and family might be helpful. Discussing your feelings with someone else could prove beneficial. If you feel like you need someone to talk to, ask your doctor for a referral to a social worker or psychologist. These are additional sources of help. Speak with your rabbi, pastor, or other spiritual advisor. Joining a support group, whether local or virtual, can be beneficial as it can provide a different viewpoint and a deeper understanding of what you're going through from other cancer sufferers.

THE END